Healing scriptures coloring book

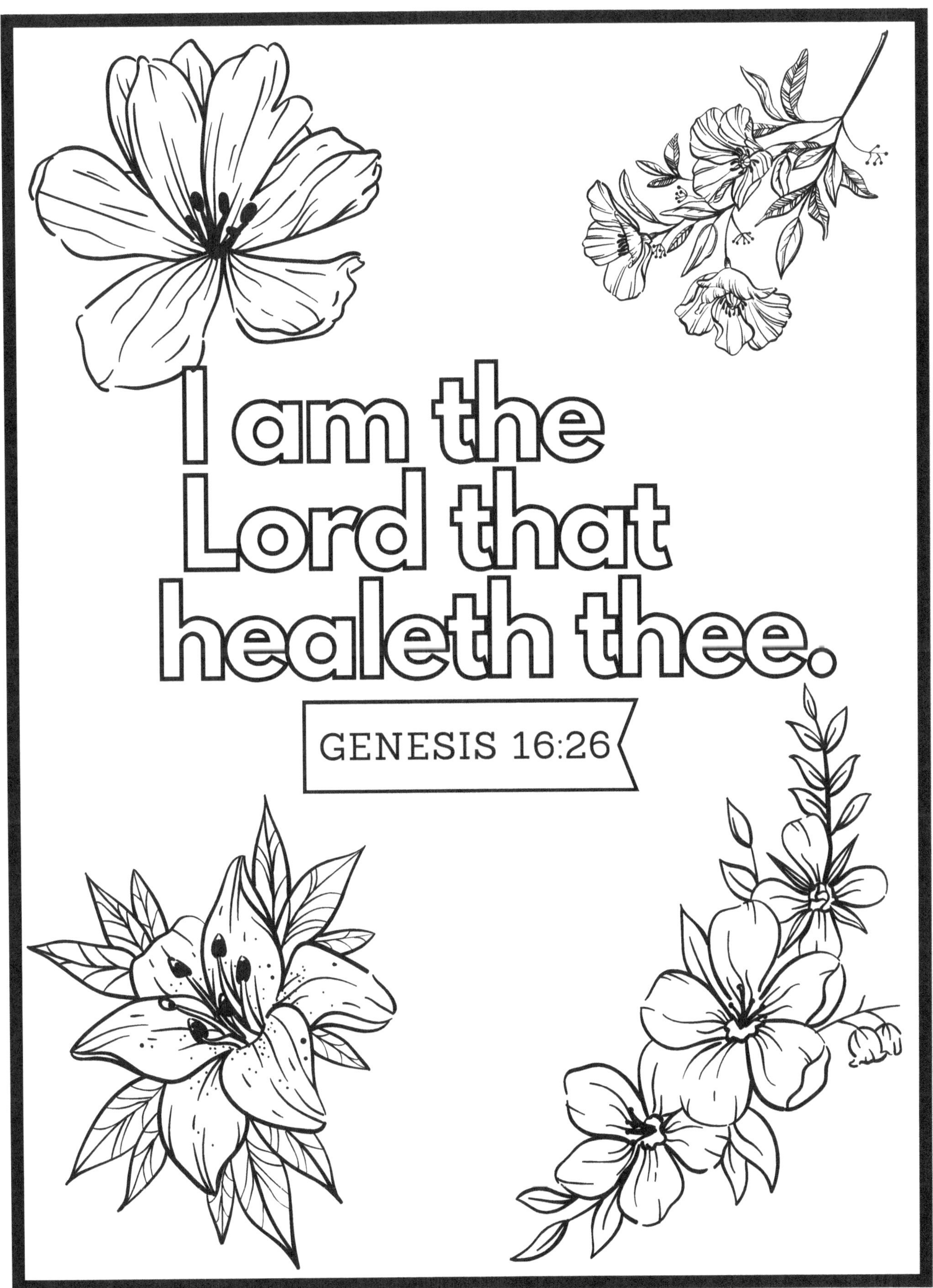

I am the Lord that healeth thee.
GENESIS 16:26

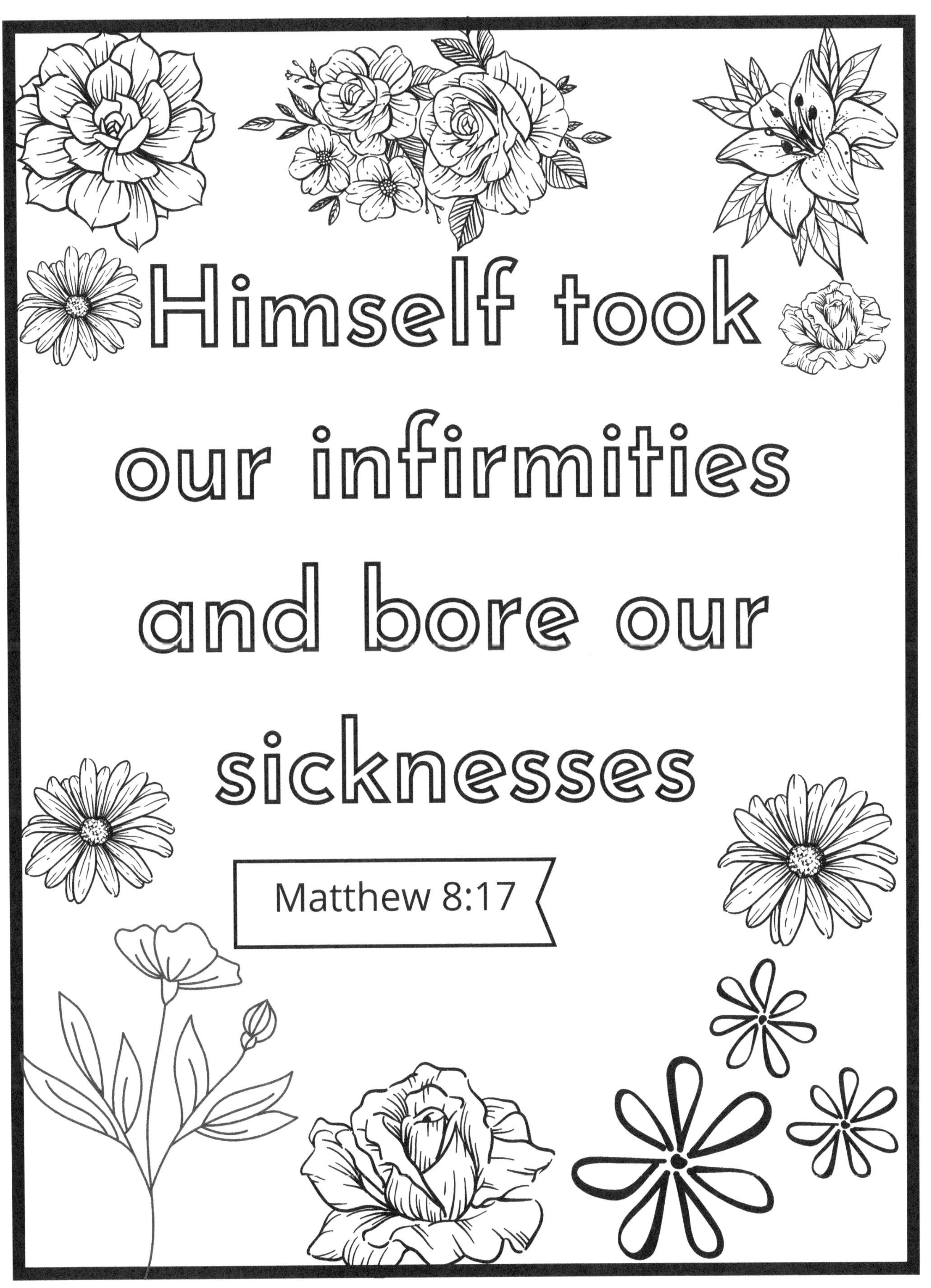
Himself took our infirmities and bore our sicknesses
Matthew 8:17

But I will restore you to health and heal
your wounds, declares the LORD.
Jeremiah 30:17

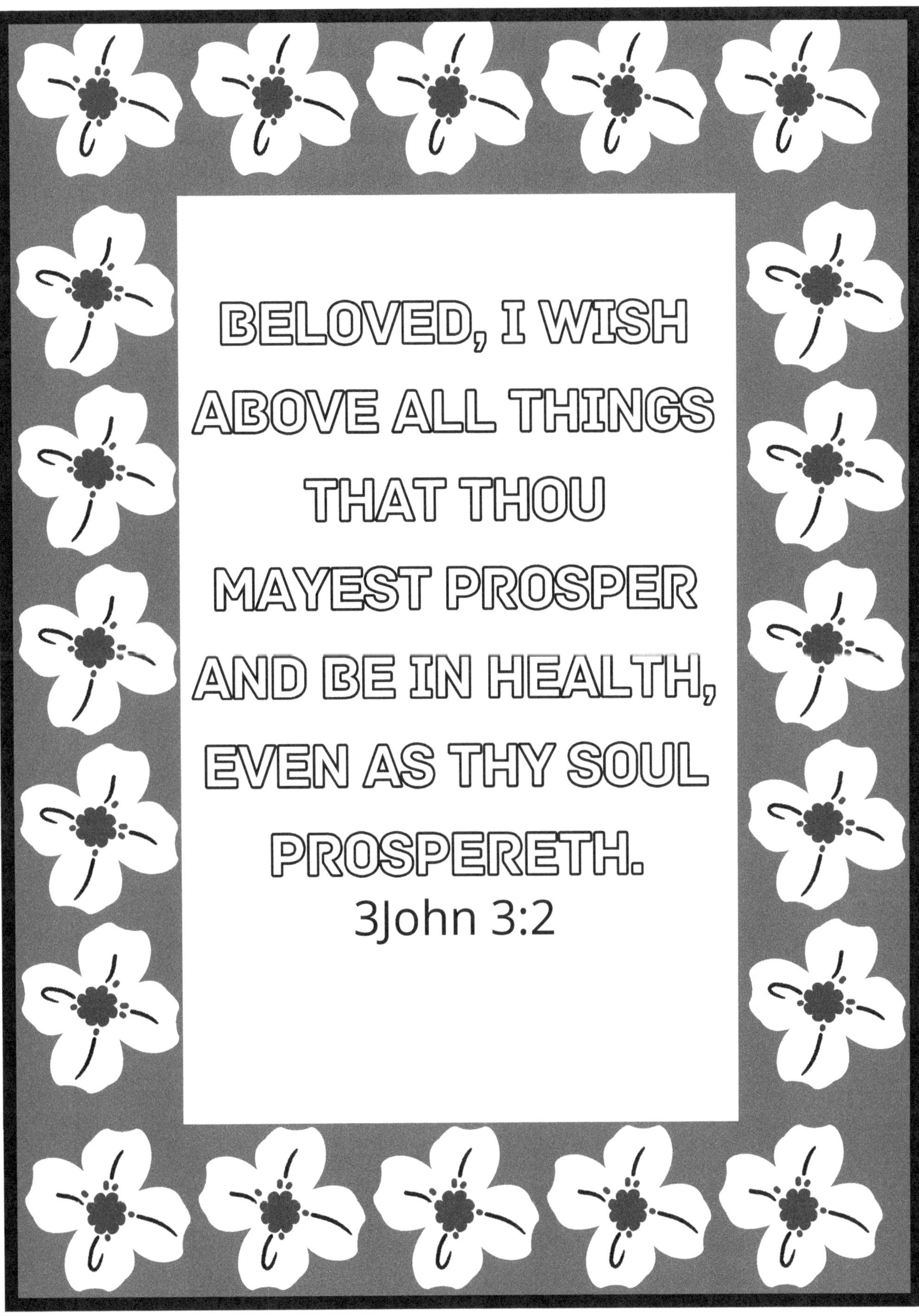
BELOVED, I WISH
ABOVE ALL THINGS
THAT THOU
MAYEST PROSPER
AND BE IN HEALTH,
EVEN AS THY SOUL
PROSPERETH.
3John 3:2

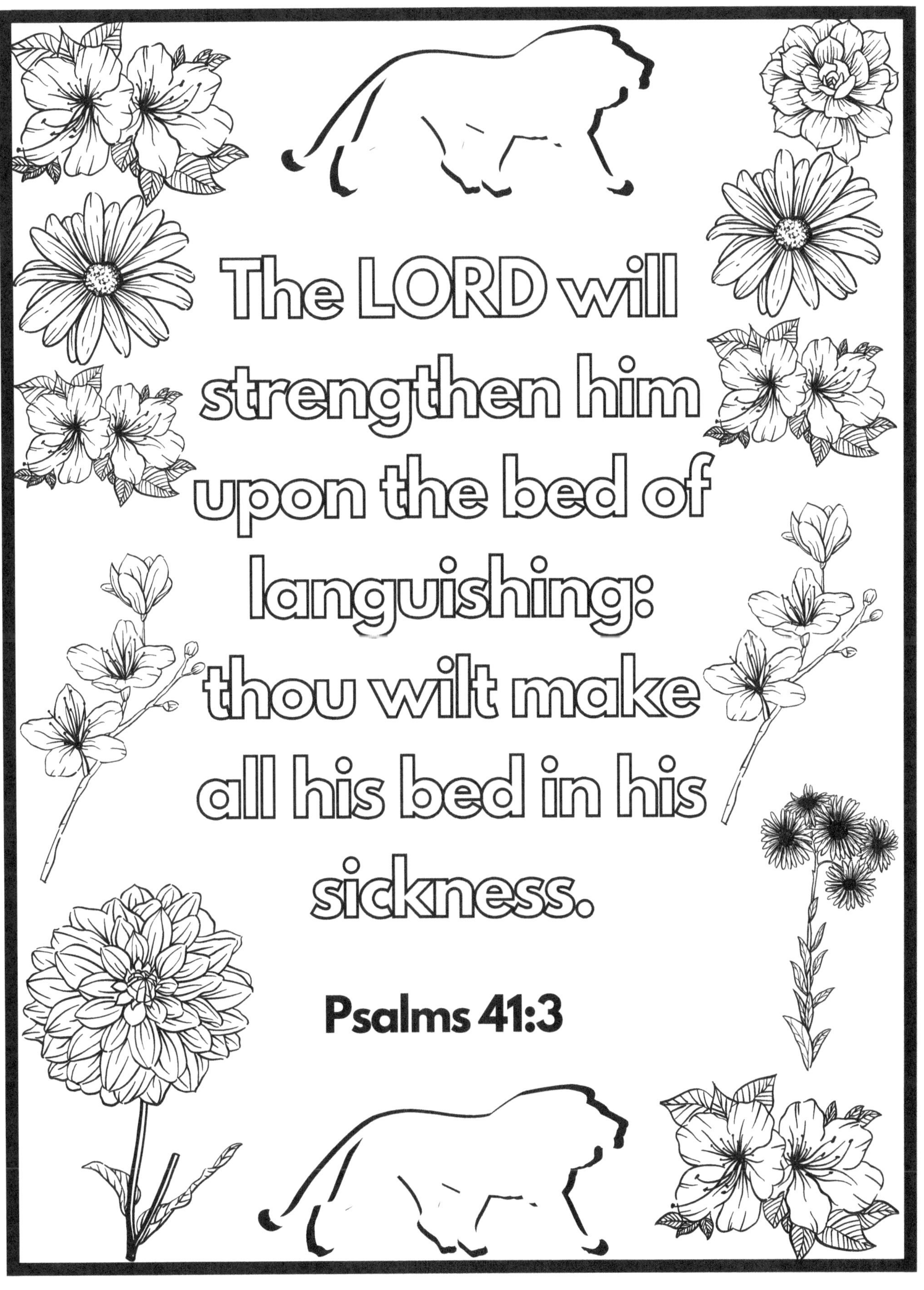

The LORD will strengthen him upon the bed of languishing: thou wilt make all his bed in his sickness.
Psalms 41:3

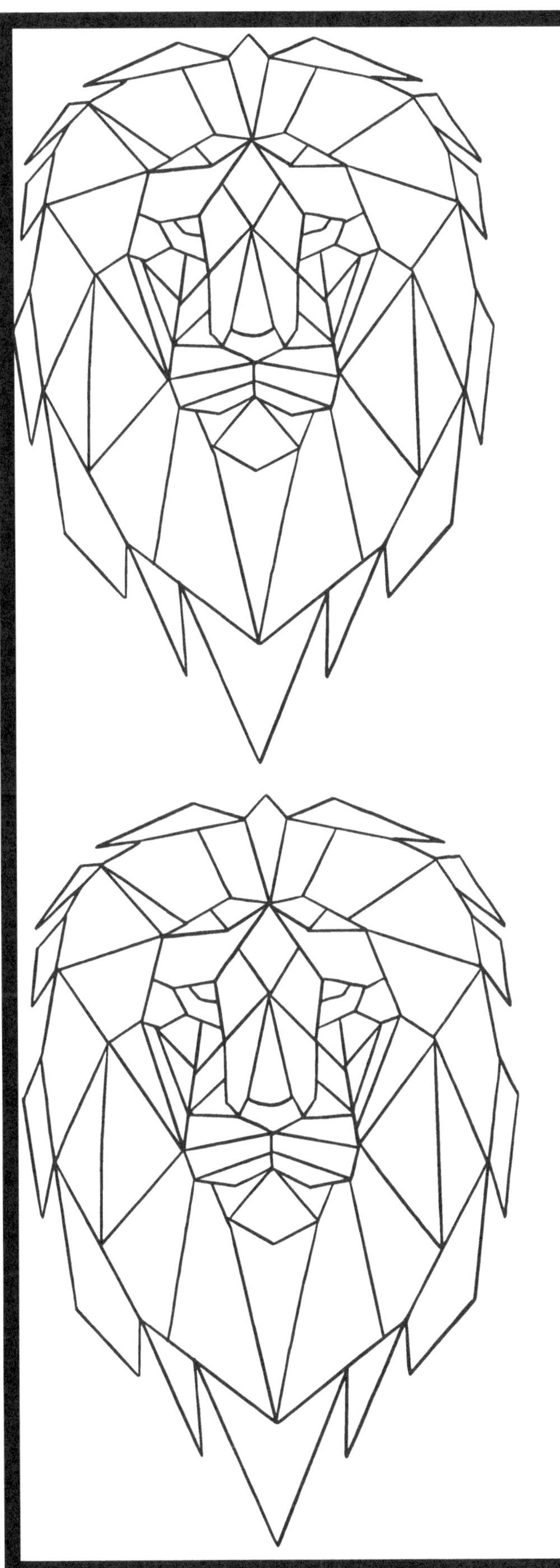

Pray one for another, that ye may be healed.

James 5:16

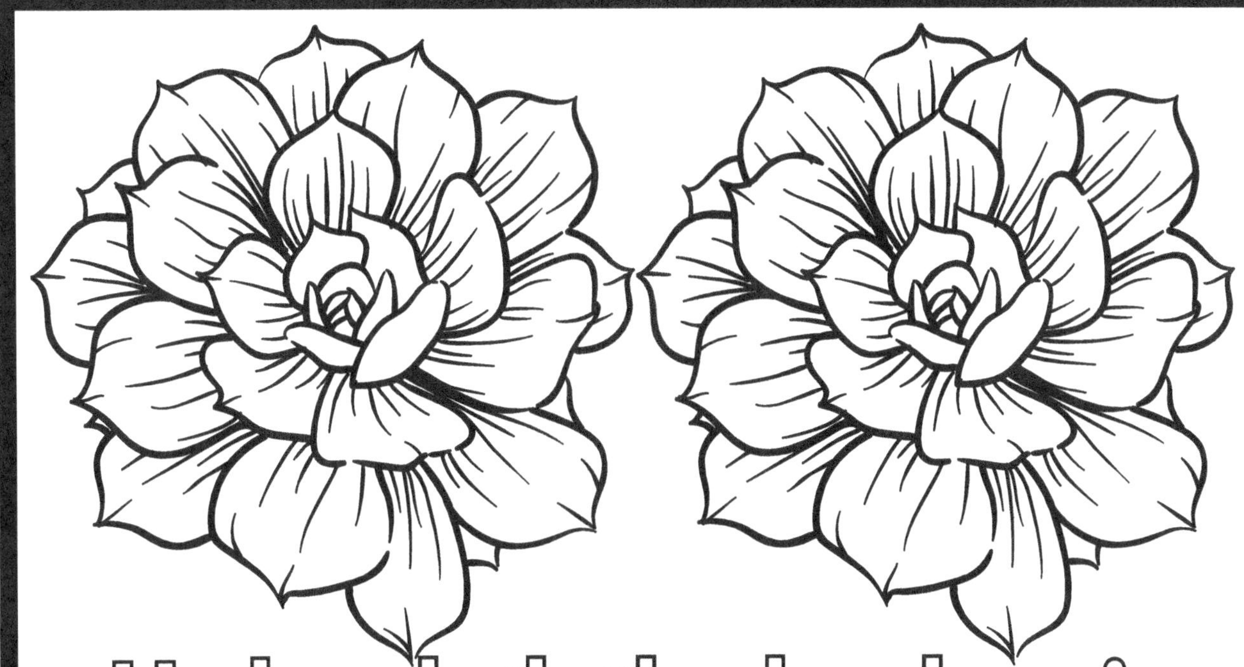

He healeth the broken in heart, and bindeth up their wounds.

Psalms 147:3

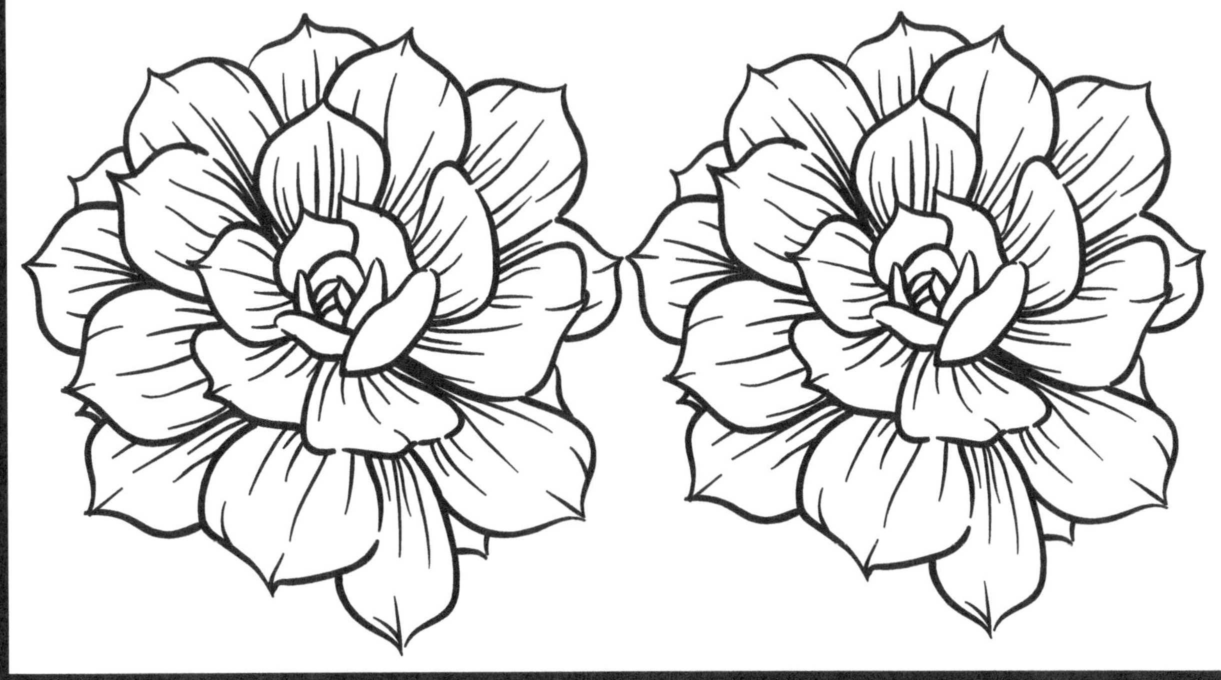

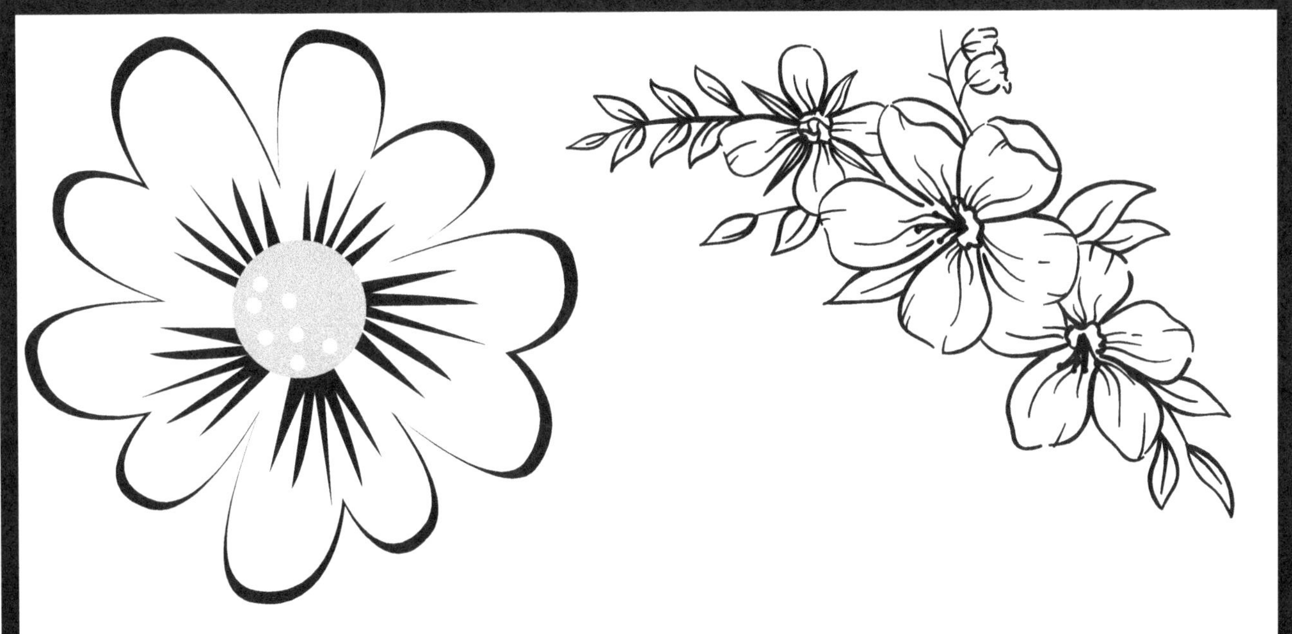

A merry heart doeth good like a medicine: but a broken spirit drieth the bones.

Proverbs 17:22

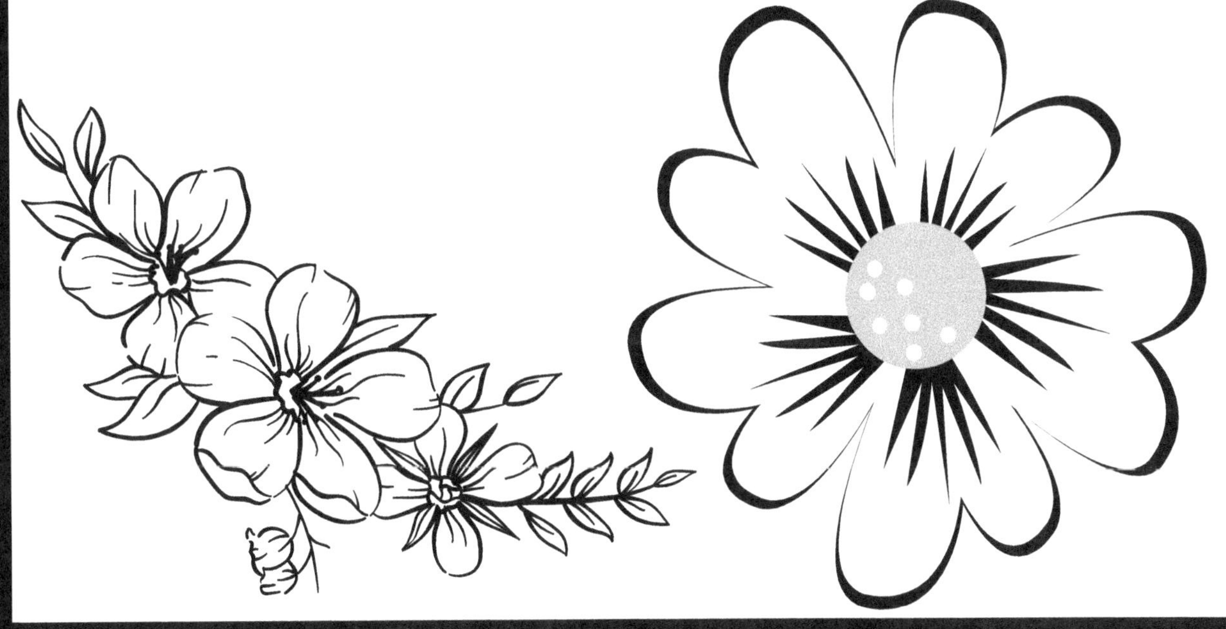

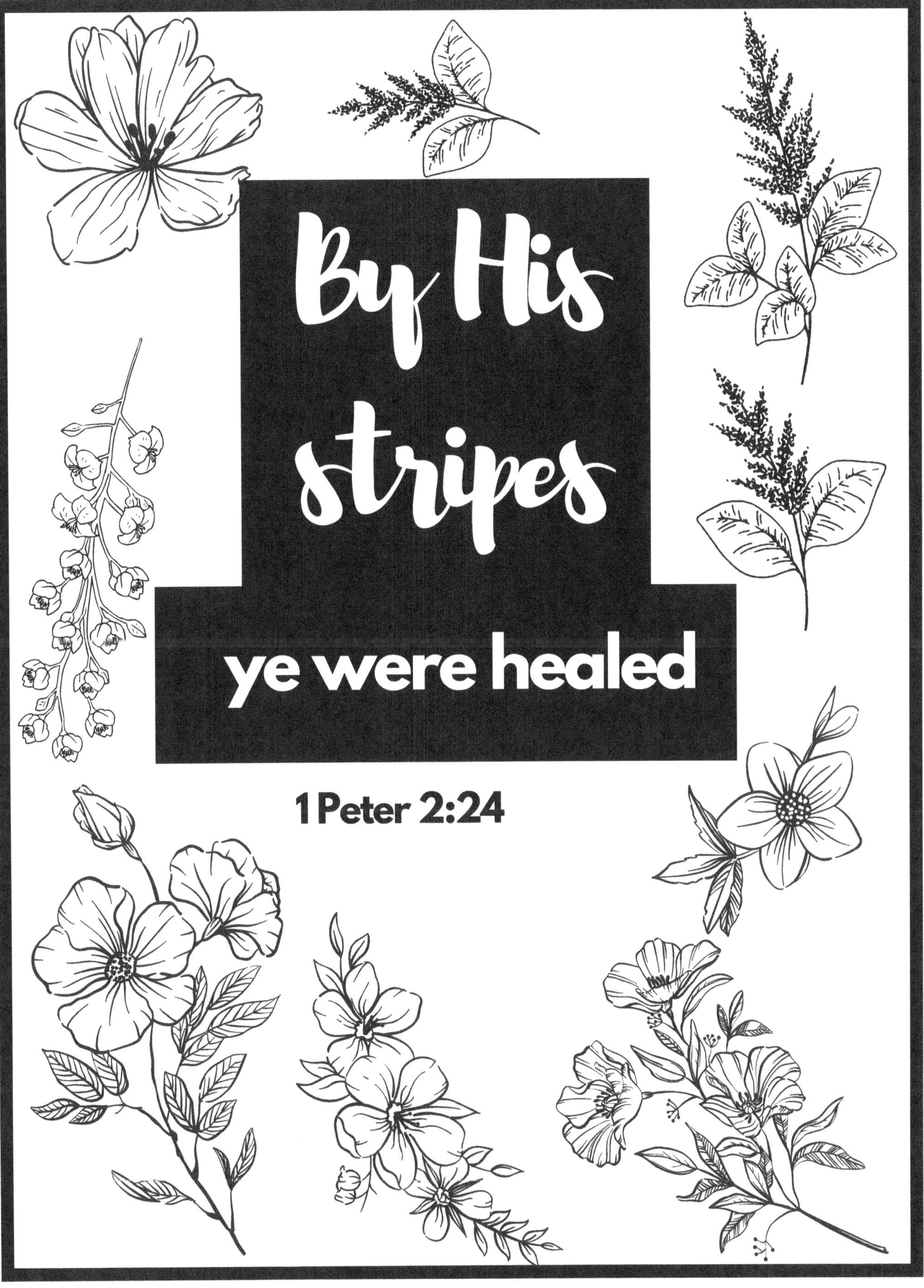

By His
stripes
ye were healed
1 Peter 2:24

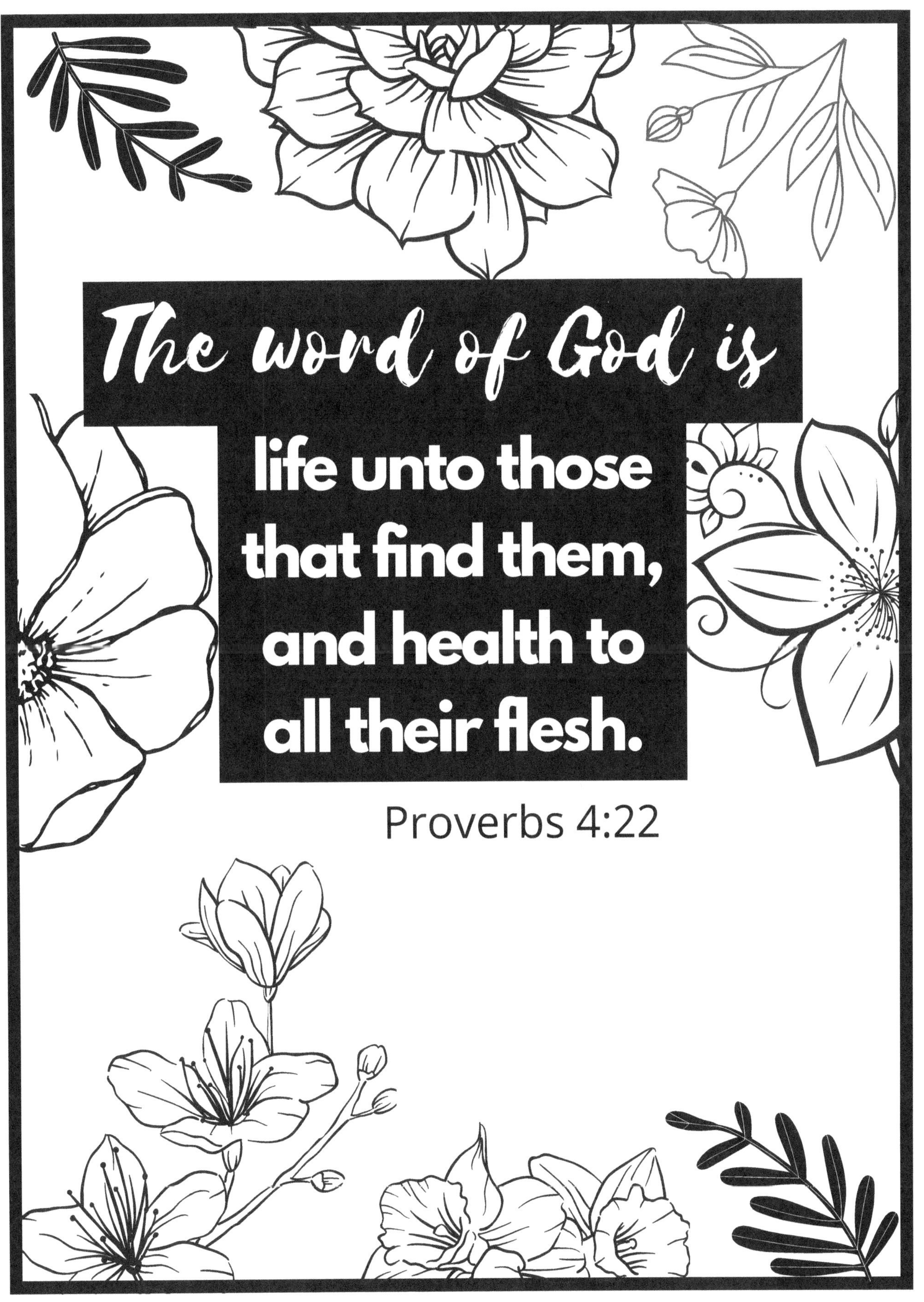
The word of God is
life unto those
that find them,
and health to
all their flesh.
Proverbs 4:22

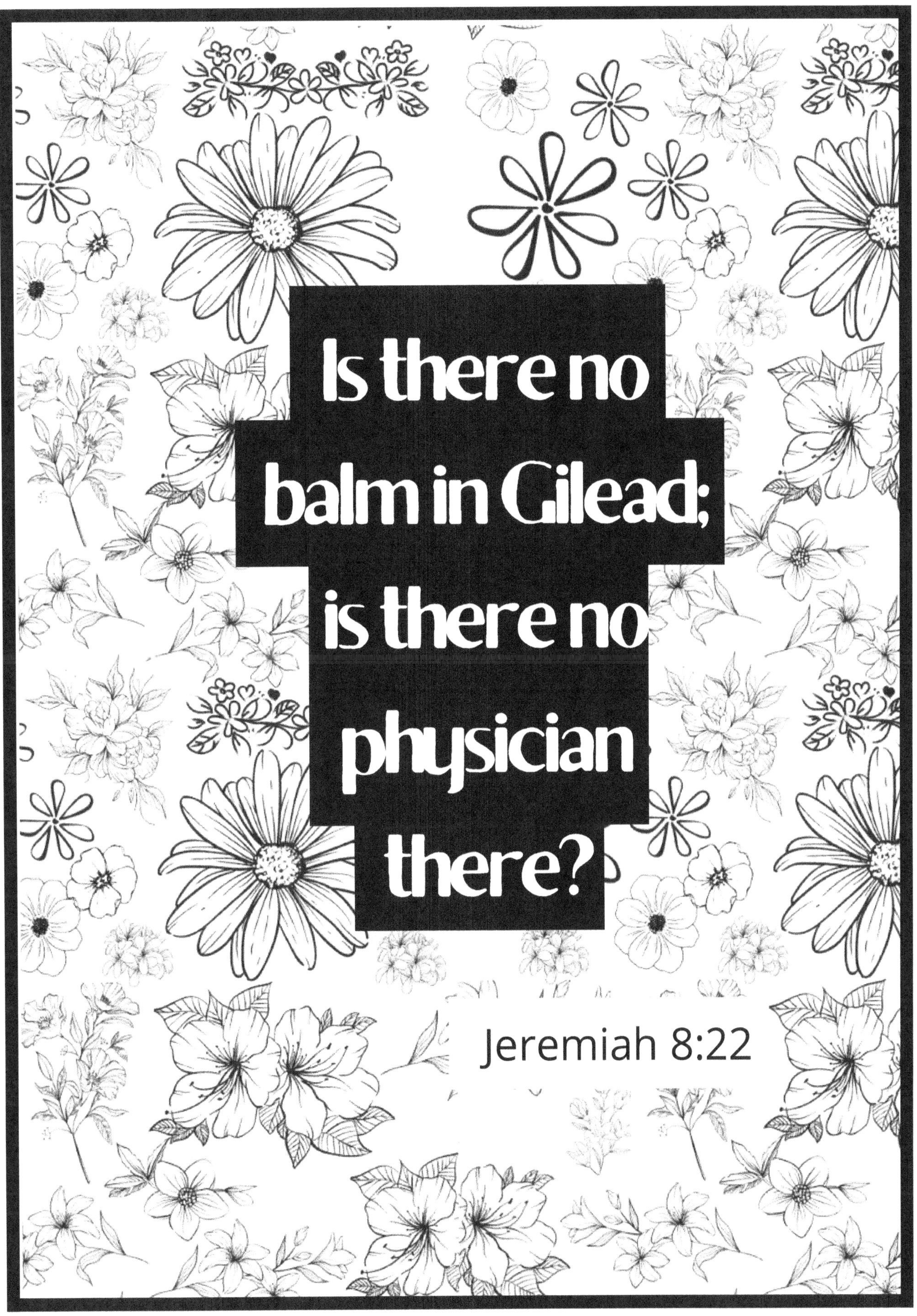

Is there no balm in Gilead; is there no physician there?

Jeremiah 8:22

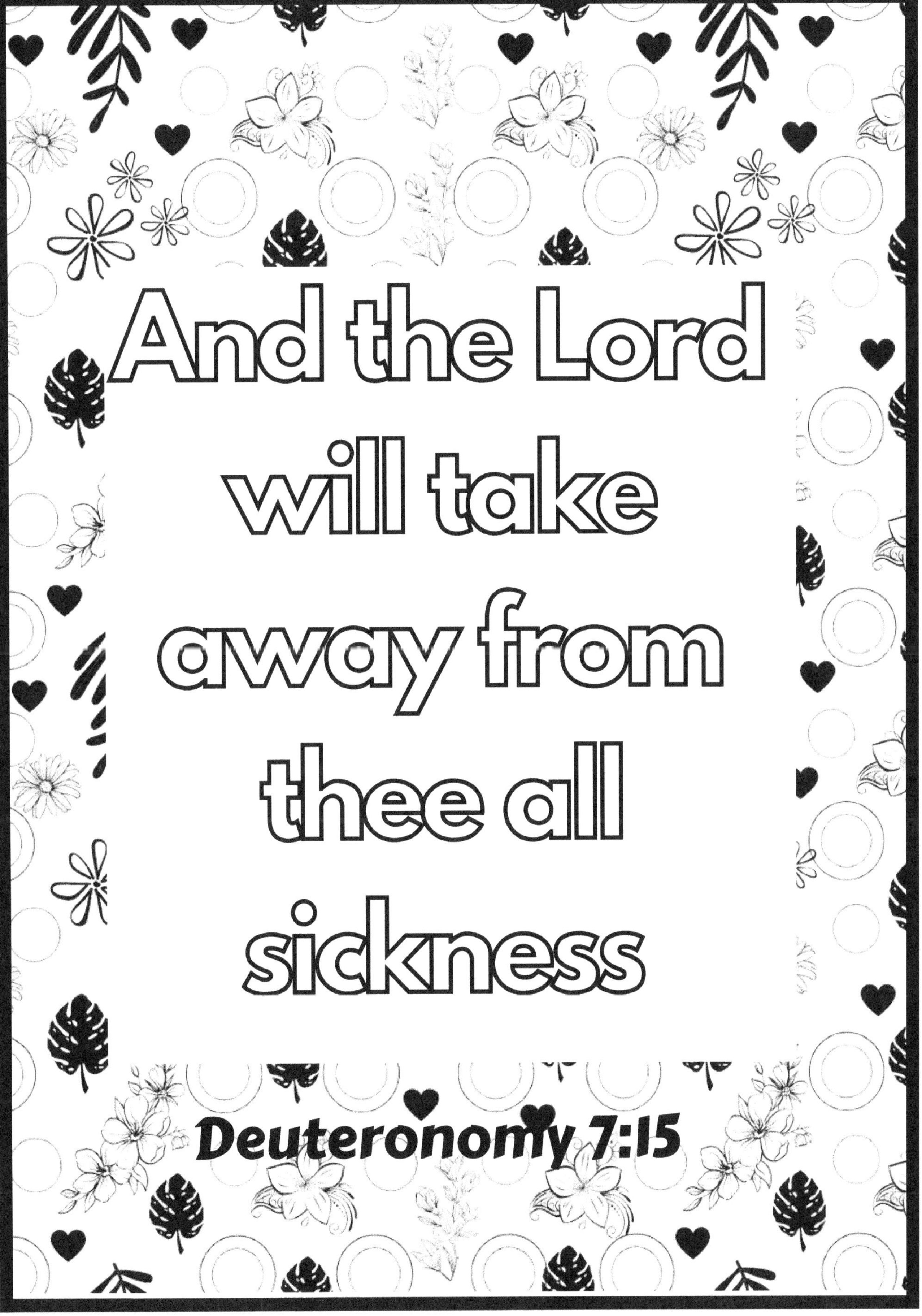

And the Lord will take away from thee all sickness
Deuteronomy 7:15

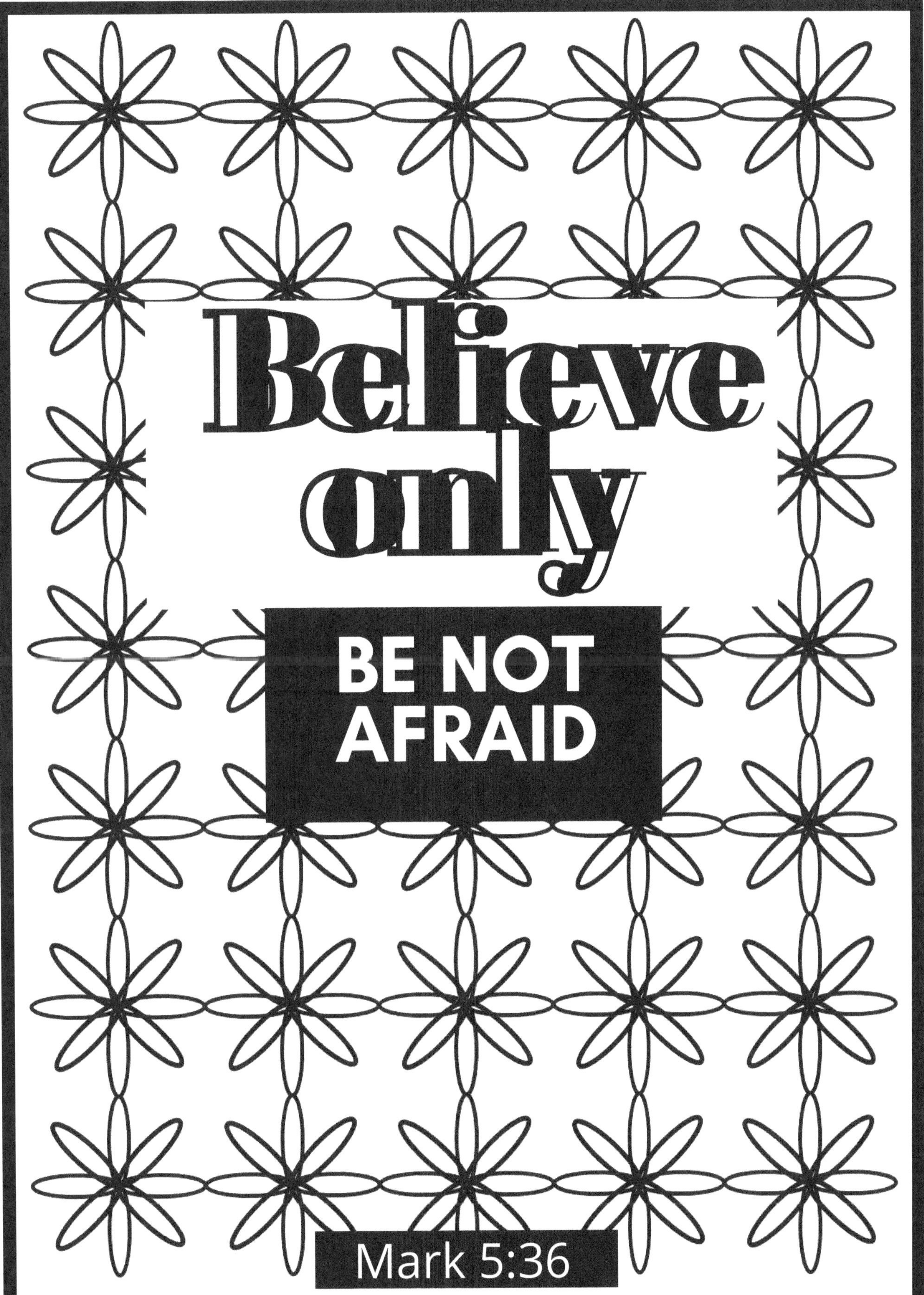
Believe only
BE NOT
AFRAID
Mark 5:36

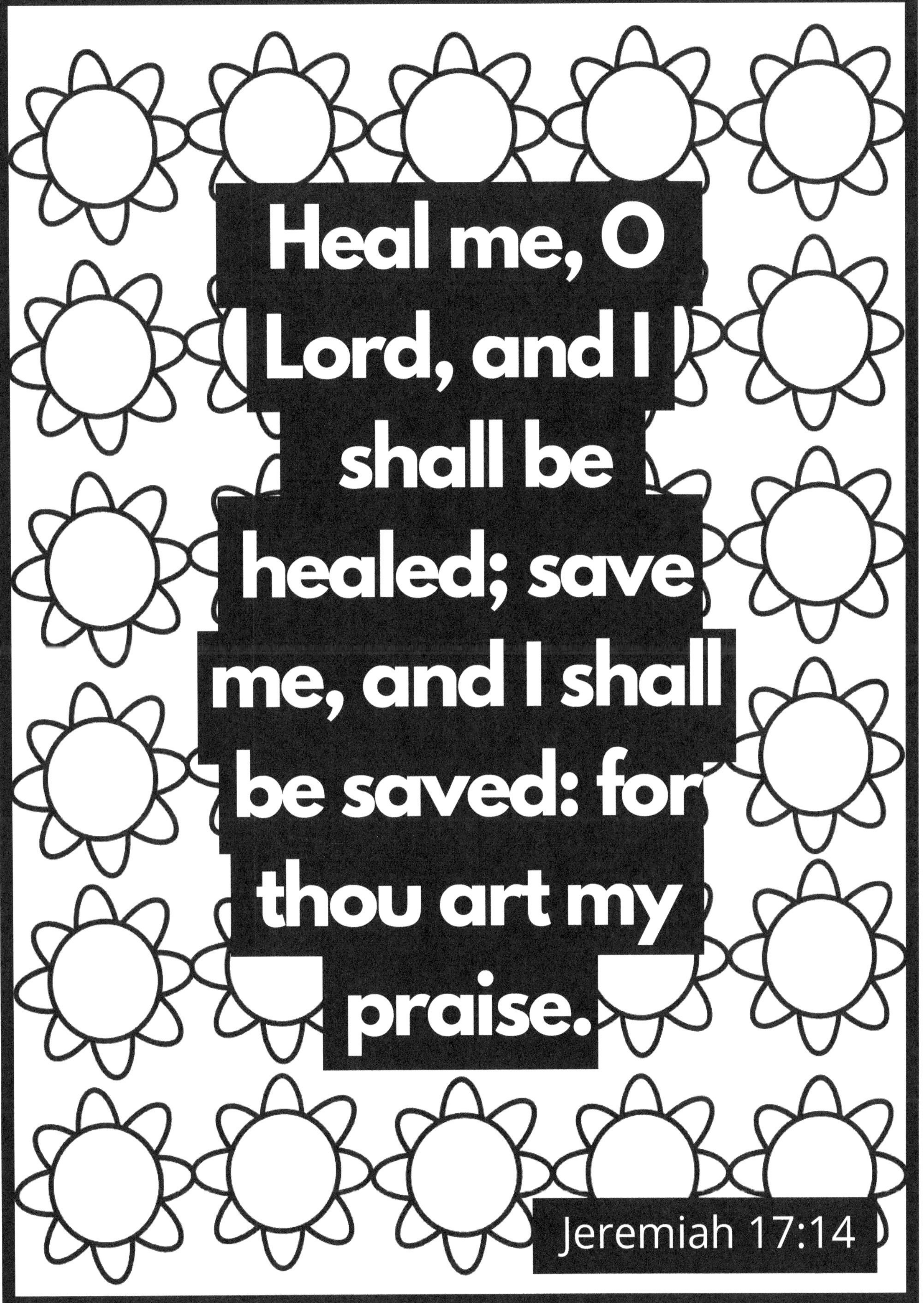

Heal me, O Lord, and I shall be healed; save me, and I shall be saved: for thou art my praise.
Jeremiah 17:14

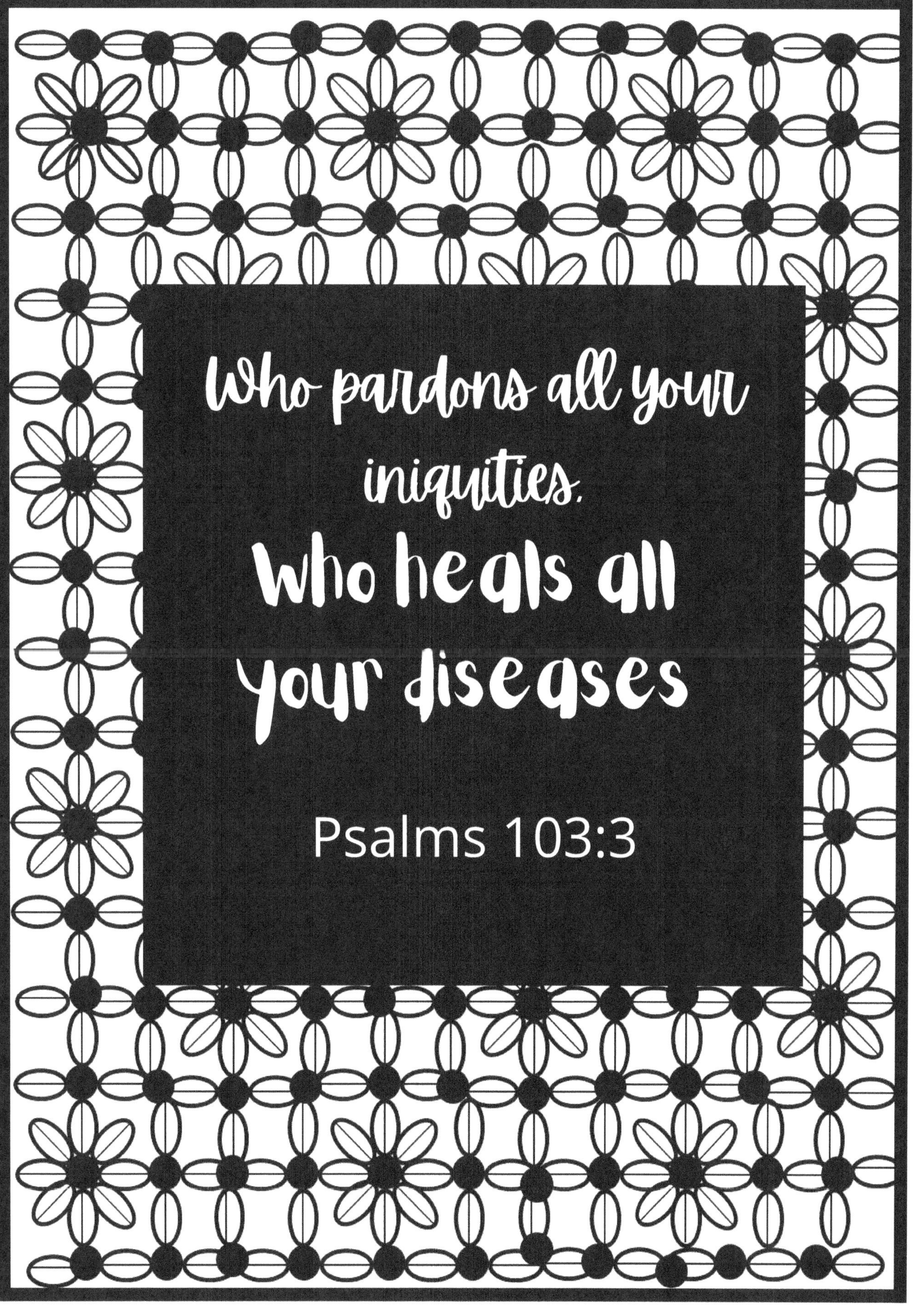

Who pardons all your iniquities,
who heals all your diseases
Psalms 103:3

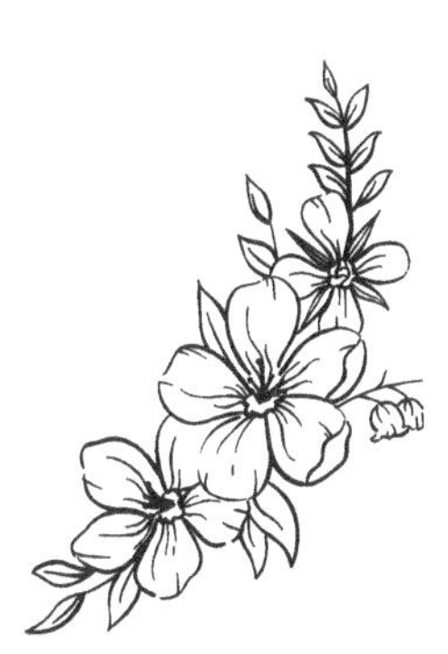
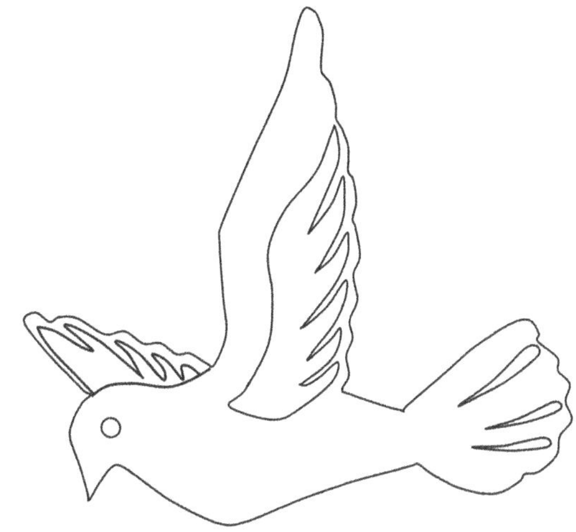

In the midst of the street of it, and on either side of the river, was there

the tree of life,

which bare

twelve manner of fruits.

and yielded her fruit every month: and the leaves of the tree were for the healing of the nations.

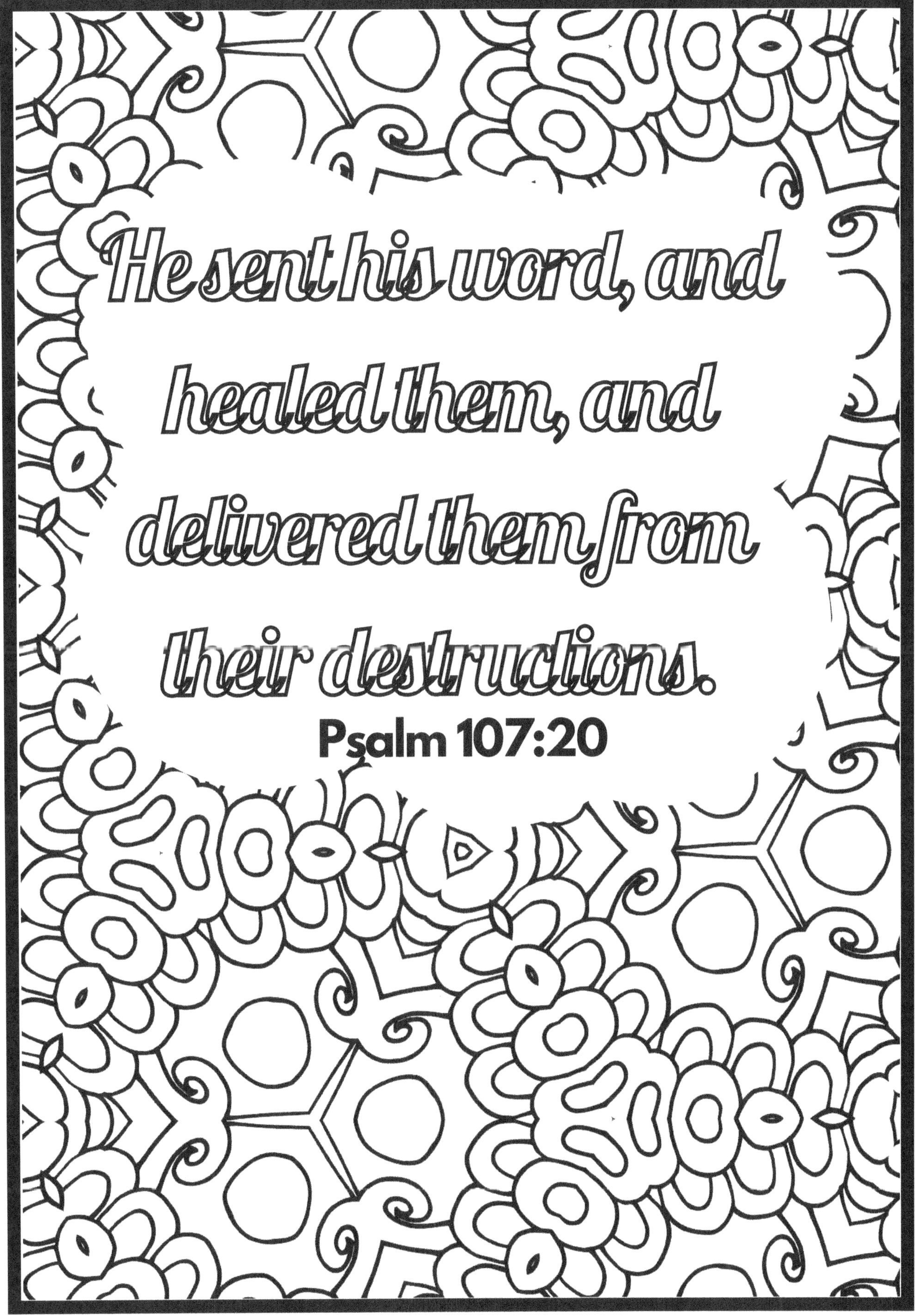

He sent his word, and healed them, and delivered them from their destructions.
Psalm 107:20

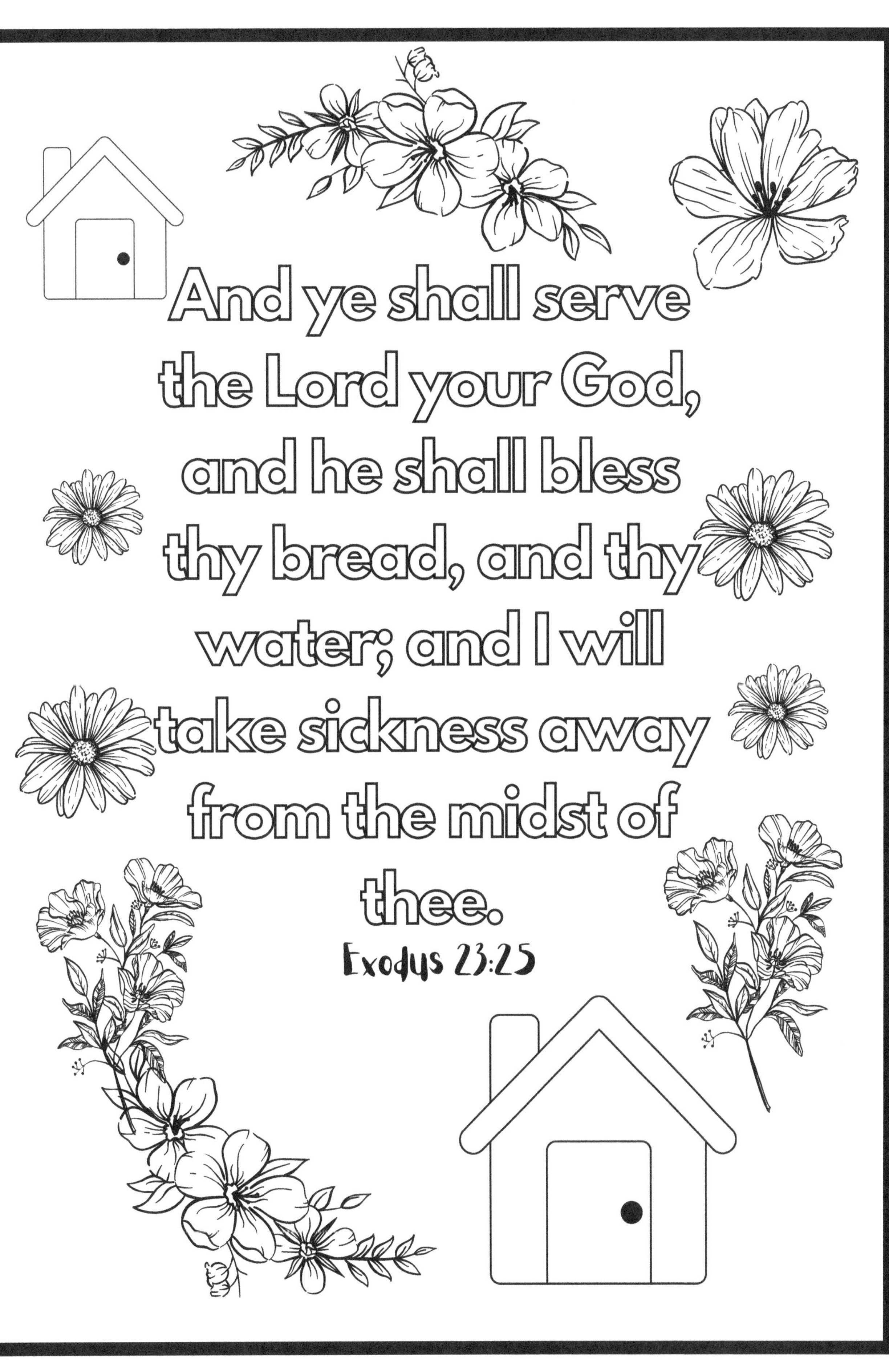

And ye shall serve the Lord your God, and he shall bless thy bread, and thy water; and I will take sickness away from the midst of thee.
Exodus 23:25

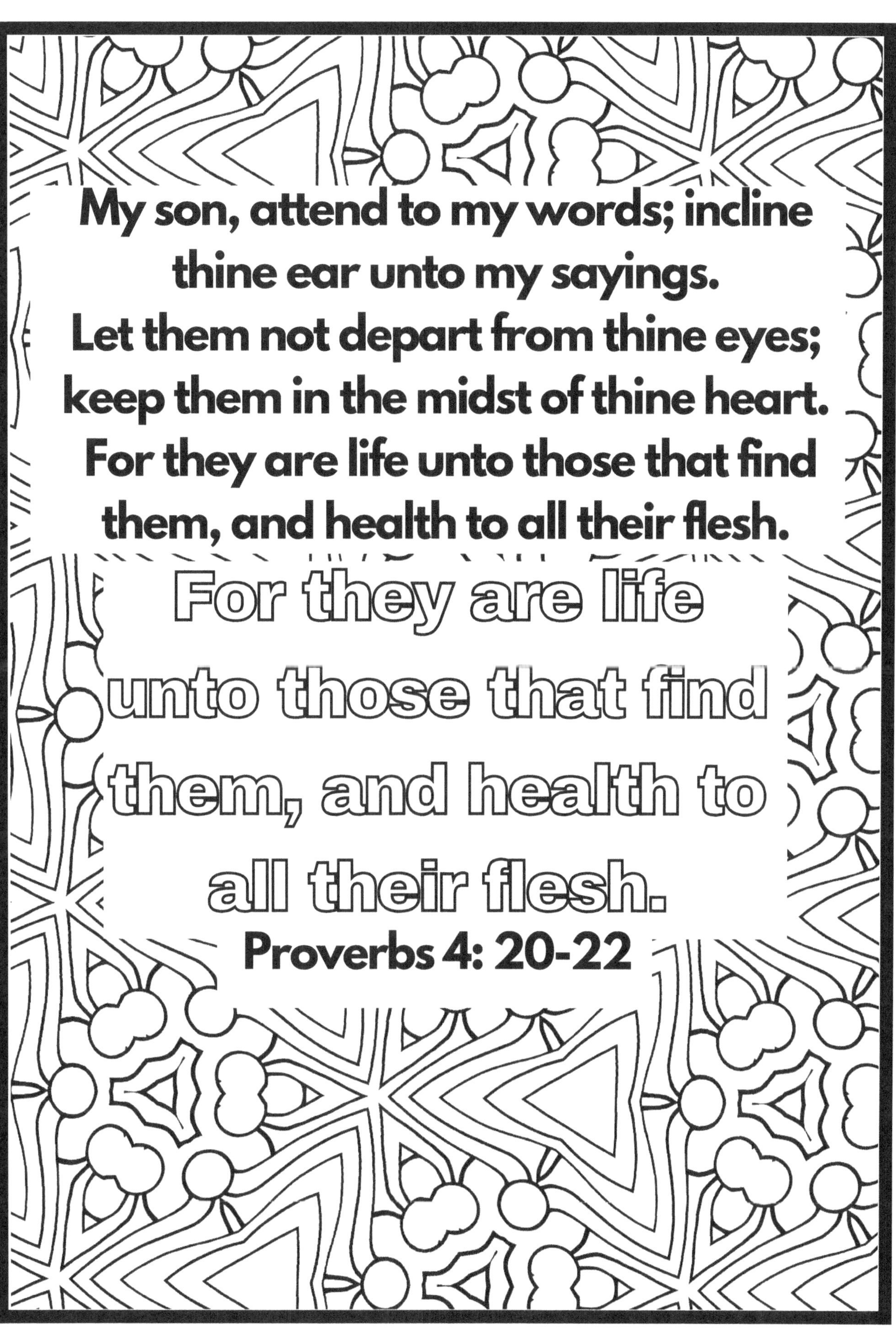
My son, attend to my words; incline thine ear unto my sayings.
Let them not depart from thine eyes; keep them in the midst of thine heart.
For they are life unto those that find them, and health to all their flesh.
For they are life unto those that find them, and health to all their flesh.
Proverbs 4: 20-22

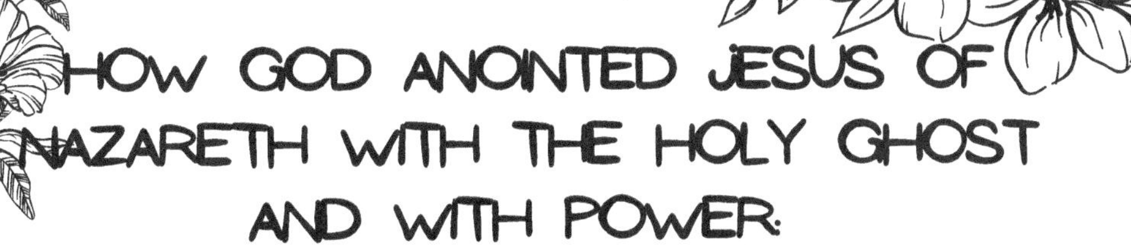

HOW GOD ANOINTED JESUS OF NAZARETH WITH THE HOLY GHOST AND WITH POWER: WHO WENT ABOUT DOING GOOD, AND HEALING ALL THAT WERE OPPRESSED OF THE DEVIL; FOR GOD WAS WITH HIM.

Act 10:38.

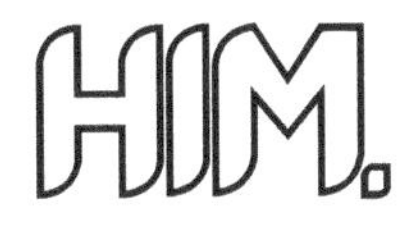

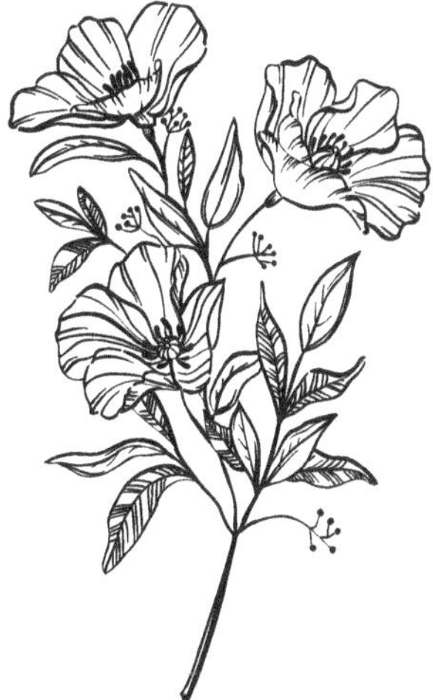

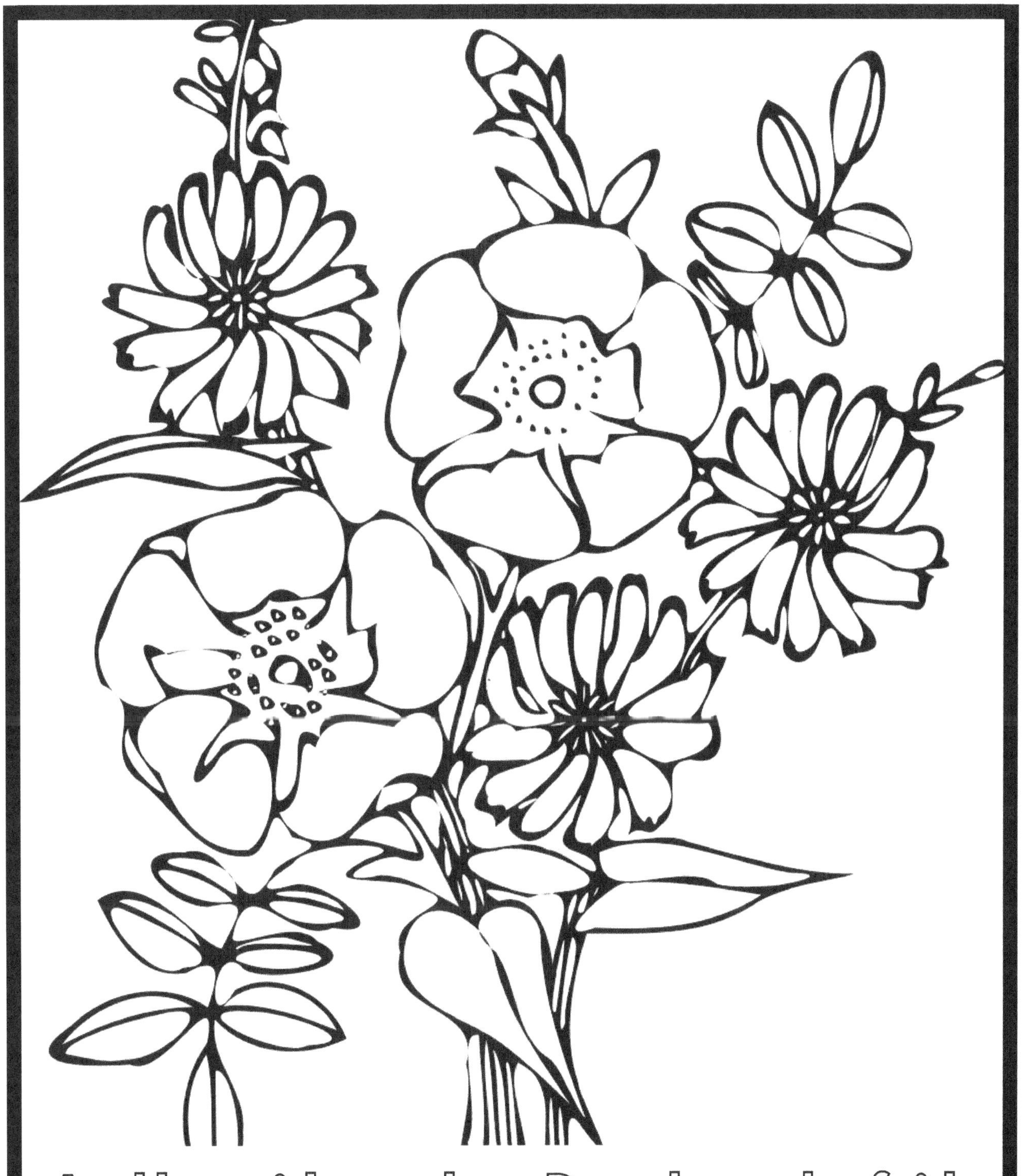

And he said unto her, Daughter, thy faith hath made thee whole; go in peace, and be whole of thy plague.

Mark 5:34

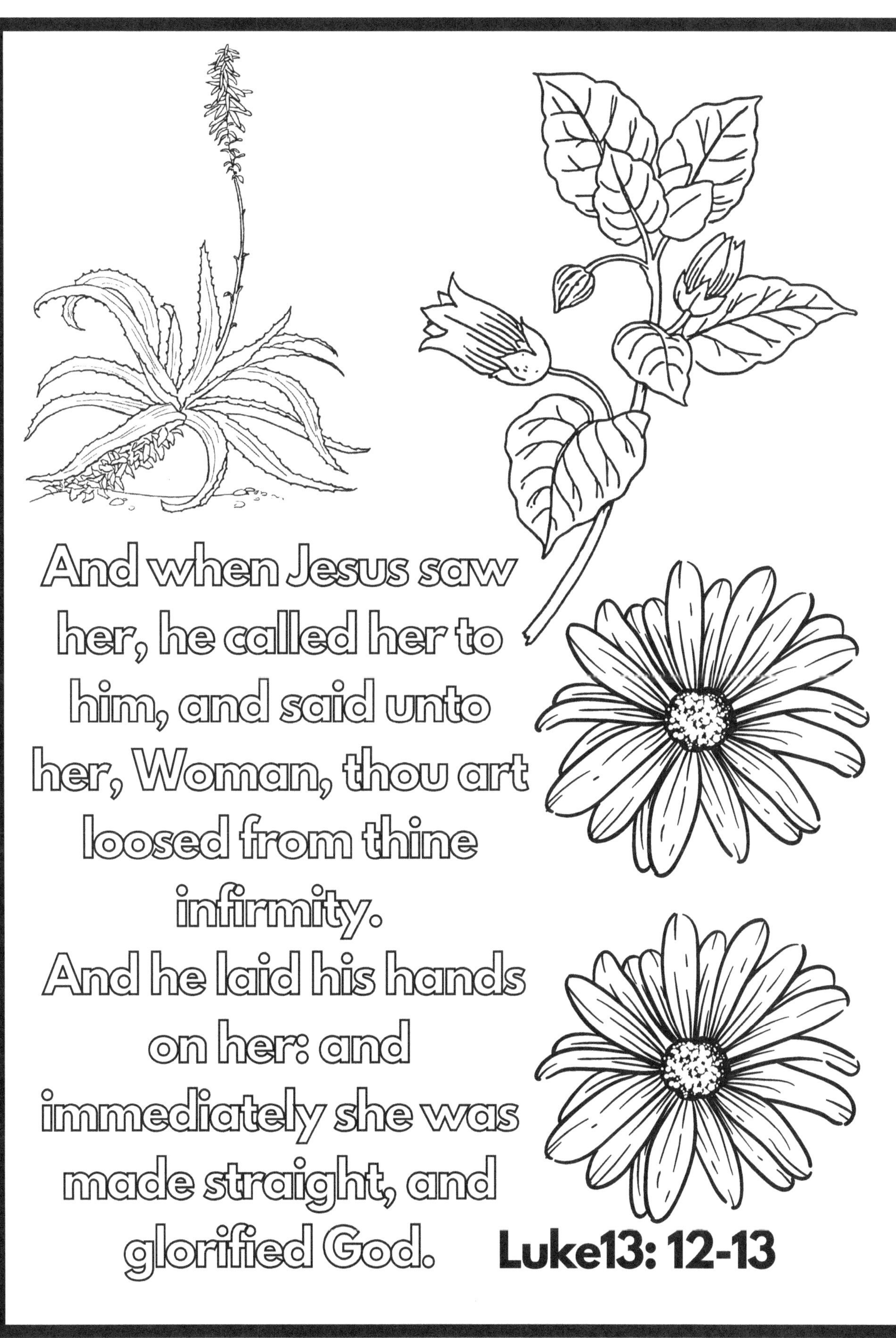

And when Jesus saw her, he called her to him, and said unto her, Woman, thou art loosed from thine infirmity.
And he laid his hands on her: and immediately she was made straight, and glorified God.
Luke13: 12-13

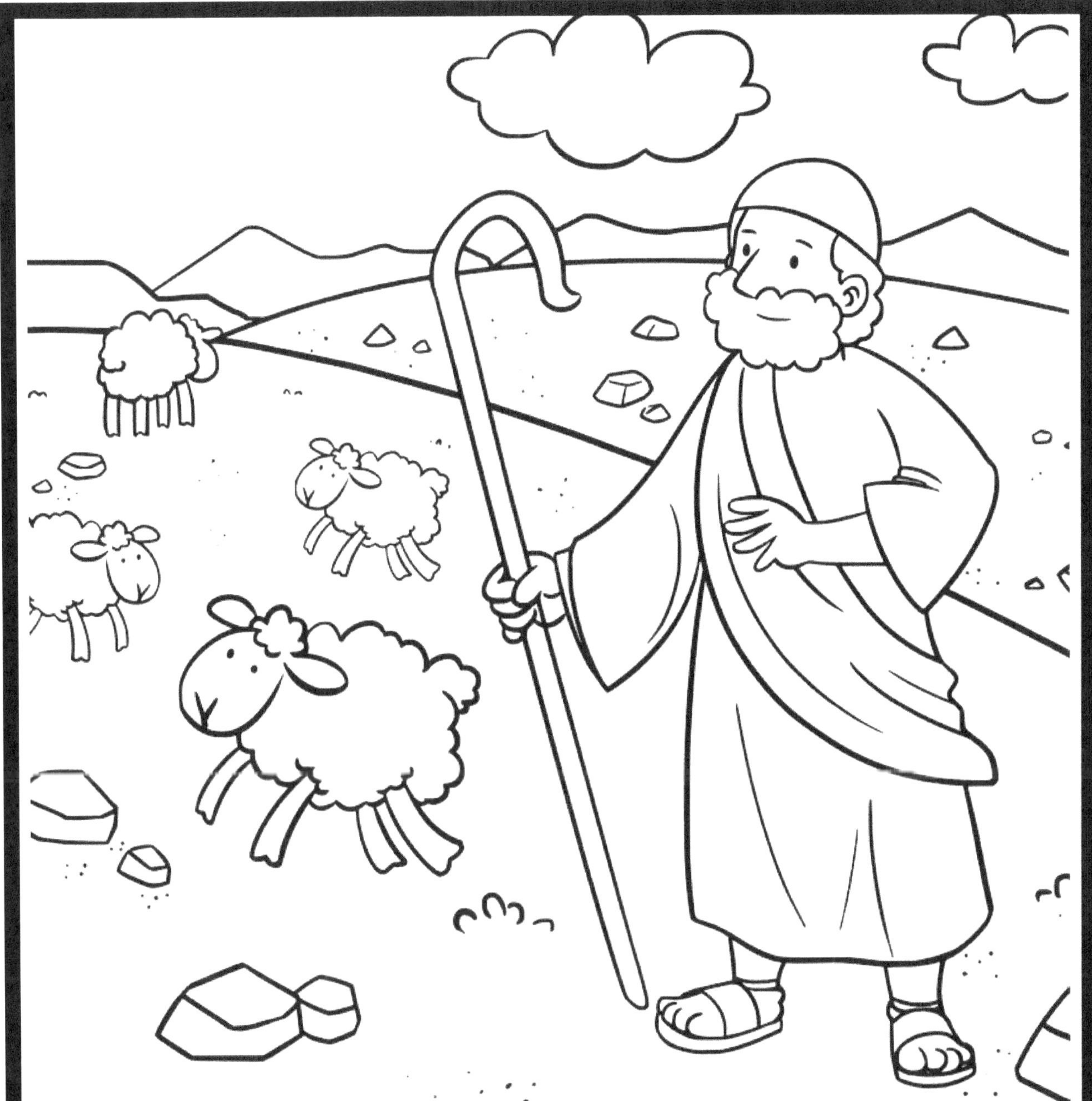

THE LORD IS MY SHEPHERD; I SHALL NOT WANT.

Psalms 23:1

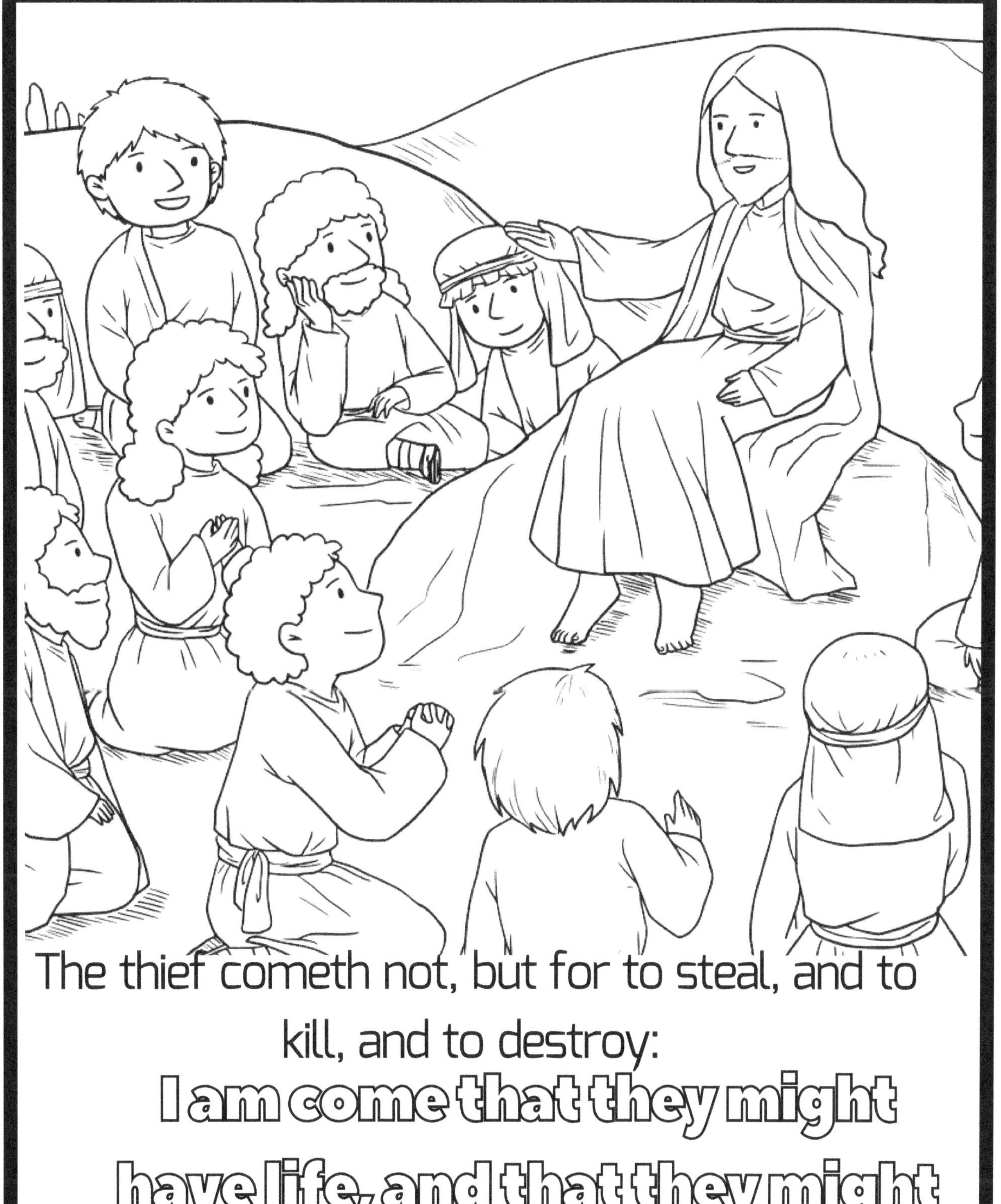

The thief cometh not, but for to steal, and to kill, and to destroy: I am come that they might have life, and that they might have it more abundantly.

John 10:10